INDEX

Name	Description	
My Profile	Name – Address – Phone Birth - Blood Type – Weight – Assistive Devices	
Medical Conditions	Basic Medical Conditions	2
Allergies	Medicine and Food Allergies	2
Emergency Contact Person	Name – Phone – Alternate Phone - Relationship	2
Medication	Name – Description - Doses	3
Surgical Procedures	Date - Procedure - Description	4
Immunizations	Name – Description - Date	4
Insurance	Insurance Type – Provider – Contact – Address – Policy Number	5
Doctor/Specialist Visits	Doctor's Name – Office – Date & Time – Reason for Visit – Questions(s) to Ask – Doctor's Diagnose/Feedback - Prescribed Treatment – Blood Pressure – Weight – Heartbeat – Blood Sugar – Oxygen Saturation – Temperature Tests Ordered – Test Results Prescribed Medication, Vitamins & Supplements	6-107
Notes	Space for your notes	108
Address Book	Primary Care Physiscian - Dentist - Eye Doctor - OB-Gyn – Specialists	112

MY PROFILE

Basic Information

Name:	
Phone:	
Address:	
Date of Birth:	
Blood Type:	
Height:	
Weight:	
Assistive Devices:	

Medical Conditions

Allergies

Emergency Contact Person

Name:	
Phone:	
Alternate Phone:	
Relationship:	

MEDICATION

Name	Description	Dosage

Notes:

SURGICAL PROCEDURES

Date	Procedure	Notes

IMMUNIZATIONS

Name / Description	Date

Notes

INSURANCE

Insurance type	
Insurance provider:	
Policy Number:	
Contact	
Phone	
Address	
Website	
Notes:	

Insurance type	
Insurance provider:	
Policy Number:	
Contact	
Phone	
Address	
Website	
Notes	

Insurance type	
Insurance provider:	
Policy Number:	
Contact	
Phone	
Address	
Website	
Notes	

DOCTOR VISITS

Doctor's Name	
Doctor's Office	
Telephone	
Date	Time
Reason for Visit	
Question(s) to Ask	
Doctor's Diagnose/ Feedback	
Prescribed Treatment	

Weight:	Blood Pressure:
Heart Rate:	Blood Sugar:
Temperature:	Oxygen Saturation:

DOCTOR VISITS

Test Ordered	Test Results

Prescription(s), Vitamins & Supplements

Name	Dosage	Duration

Notes:

DOCTOR VISITS

Doctor's Name	
Doctor's Office	
Telephone	
Date	Time
Reason for Visit	
Question(s) to Ask	
Doctor's Diagnose/ Feedback	
Prescribed Treatment	

Weight:	Blood Pressure:
Heart Rate:	Blood Sugar:
Temperature:	Oxygen Saturation:

DOCTOR VISITS

Test Ordered	Test Results

Prescription(s), Vitamins & Supplements

Name	Dosage	Duration

Notes:

DOCTOR VISITS

Doctor's Name	
Doctor's Office	
Telephone	
Date	Time
Reason for Visit	
Question(s) to Ask	
Doctor's Diagnose/ Feedback	
Prescribed Treatment	

Weight:	Blood Pressure:
Heart Rate:	Blood Sugar:
Temperature:	Oxygen Saturation:

DOCTOR VISITS

Test Ordered	Test Results

Prescription(s), Vitamins & Supplements

Name	Dosage	Duration

Notes:

DOCTOR VISITS

Doctor's Name	
Doctor's Office	
Telephone	
Date	

Date		Time	

Reason for Visit	
Question(s) to Ask	
Doctor's Diagnose/ Feedback	
Prescribed Treatment	

Weight:		Blood Pressure:	
Heart Rate:		Blood Sugar:	
Temperature:		Oxygen Saturation:	

DOCTOR VISITS

Test Ordered	Test Results

Prescription(s), Vitamins & Supplements

Name	Dosage	Duration

Notes:

DOCTOR VISITS

Doctor's Name	
Doctor's Office	
Telephone	
Date	Time
Reason for Visit	
Question(s) to Ask	
Doctor's Diagnose/ Feedback	
Prescribed Treatment	

Weight:	Blood Pressure:
Heart Rate:	Blood Sugar:
Temperature:	Oxygen Saturation:

DOCTOR VISITS

Test Ordered	Test Results

Prescription(s), Vitamins & Supplements

Name	Dosage	Duration

Notes:

DOCTOR VISITS

Doctor's Name	
Doctor's Office	
Telephone	
Date	Time
Reason for Visit	
Question(s) to Ask	
Doctor's Diagnose/ Feedback	
Prescribed Treatment	

Weight:	Blood Pressure:
Heart Rate:	Blood Sugar:
Temperature:	Oxygen Saturation:

DOCTOR VISITS

Test Ordered	Test Results

Prescription(s), Vitamins & Supplements

Name	Dosage	Duration

Notes:

DOCTOR VISITS

Doctor's Name	
Doctor's Office	
Telephone	
Date	Time
Reason for Visit	
Question(s) to Ask	
Doctor's Diagnose/ Feedback	
Prescribed Treatment	

Weight:	Blood Pressure:
Heart Rate:	Blood Sugar:
Temperature:	Oxygen Saturation:

DOCTOR VISITS

Test Ordered	Test Results

Prescription(s), Vitamins & Supplements

Name	Dosage	Duration

Notes:

DOCTOR VISITS

Doctor's Name	
Doctor's Office	
Telephone	
Date	Time
Reason for Visit	
Question(s) to Ask	
Doctor's Diagnose/ Feedback	
Prescribed Treatment	

Weight:	Blood Pressure:
Heart Rate:	Blood Sugar:
Temperature:	Oxygen Saturation:

DOCTOR VISITS

Test Ordered	Test Results

Prescription(s), Vitamins & Supplements

Name	Dosage	Duration

Notes:

DOCTOR VISITS

Doctor's Name	
Doctor's Office	
Telephone	
Date	Time
Reason for Visit	
Question(s) to Ask	
Doctor's Diagnose/ Feedback	
Prescribed Treatment	

Weight:	Blood Pressure:
Heart Rate:	Blood Sugar:
Temperature:	Oxygen Saturation:

DOCTOR VISITS

Test Ordered	Test Results

Prescription(s), Vitamins & Supplements

Name	Dosage	Duration

Notes:

DOCTOR VISITS

Doctor's Name	
Doctor's Office	
Telephone	

Date		Time	

Reason for Visit	
Question(s) to Ask	
Doctor's Diagnose/ Feedback	
Prescribed Treatment	

Weight:		Blood Pressure:	
Heart Rate:		Blood Sugar:	
Temperature:		Oxygen Saturation:	

DOCTOR VISITS

Test Ordered	Test Results

Prescription(s), Vitamins & Supplements

Name	Dosage	Duration

Notes:

DOCTOR VISITS

Doctor's Name	
Doctor's Office	
Telephone	
Date	Time
Reason for Visit	
Question(s) to Ask	
Doctor's Diagnose/ Feedback	
Prescribed Treatment	

Weight:	Blood Pressure:
Heart Rate:	Blood Sugar:
Temperature:	Oxygen Saturation:

DOCTOR VISITS

Test Ordered	Test Results

Prescription(s), Vitamins & Supplements

Name	Dosage	Duration

Notes:

DOCTOR VISITS

Doctor's Name	
Doctor's Office	
Telephone	
Date	Time
Reason for Visit	
Question(s) to Ask	
Doctor's Diagnose/ Feedback	
Prescribed Treatment	

Weight:	Blood Pressure:
Heart Rate:	Blood Sugar:
Temperature:	Oxygen Saturation:

DOCTOR VISITS

Test Ordered	Test Results

Prescription(s), Vitamins & Supplements

Name	Dosage	Duration

Notes:

DOCTOR VISITS

Doctor's Name	
Doctor's Office	
Telephone	

Date		Time	

Reason for Visit	
Question(s) to Ask	
Doctor's Diagnose/ Feedback	
Prescribed Treatment	

Weight:	Blood Pressure:
Heart Rate:	Blood Sugar:
Temperature:	Oxygen Saturation:

DOCTOR VISITS

Test Ordered	Test Results

Prescription(s), Vitamins & Supplements

Name	Dosage	Duration

Notes:

DOCTOR VISITS

Doctor's Name	
Doctor's Office	
Telephone	
Date	Time
Reason for Visit	
Question(s) to Ask	
Doctor's Diagnose/ Feedback	
Prescribed Treatment	

Weight:	Blood Pressure:
Heart Rate:	Blood Sugar:
Temperature:	Oxygen Saturation:

DOCTOR VISITS

Test Ordered	Test Results

Prescription(s), Vitamins & Supplements

Name	Dosage	Duration

Notes:

DOCTOR VISITS

Doctor's Name	
Doctor's Office	
Telephone	

Date		Time	

Reason for Visit	
Question(s) to Ask	
Doctor's Diagnose/ Feedback	
Prescribed Treatment	

Weight:		Blood Pressure:	
Heart Rate:		Blood Sugar:	
Temperature:		Oxygen Saturation:	

DOCTOR VISITS

Test Ordered	Test Results

Prescription(s), Vitamins & Supplements

Name	Dosage	Duration

Notes:

DOCTOR VISITS

Doctor's Name	
Doctor's Office	
Telephone	
Date	Time
Reason for Visit	
Question(s) to Ask	
Doctor's Diagnose/ Feedback	
Prescribed Treatment	

Weight:	Blood Pressure:
Heart Rate:	Blood Sugar:
Temperature:	Oxygen Saturation:

DOCTOR VISITS

Test Ordered	Test Results

Prescription(s), Vitamins & Supplements

Name	Dosage	Duration

Notes:

DOCTOR VISITS

Doctor's Name	
Doctor's Office	
Telephone	
Date	Time
Reason for Visit	
Question(s) to Ask	
Doctor's Diagnose/ Feedback	
Prescribed Treatment	

Weight:	Blood Pressure:
Heart Rate:	Blood Sugar:
Temperature:	Oxygen Saturation:

DOCTOR VISITS

Test Ordered	Test Results

Prescription(s), Vitamins & Supplements

Name	Dosage	Duration

Notes:

DOCTOR VISITS

Doctor's Name	
Doctor's Office	
Telephone	

Date		Time	

Reason for Visit	
Question(s) to Ask	
Doctor's Diagnose/ Feedback	
Prescribed Treatment	

Weight:		Blood Pressure:	
Heart Rate:		Blood Sugar:	
Temperature:		Oxygen Saturation:	

DOCTOR VISITS

Test Ordered	Test Results

Prescription(s), Vitamins & Supplements

Name	Dosage	Duration

Notes:

DOCTOR VISITS

Doctor's Name	
Doctor's Office	
Telephone	
Date	Time
Reason for Visit	
Question(s) to Ask	
Doctor's Diagnose/ Feedback	
Prescribed Treatment	

Weight:	Blood Pressure:
Heart Rate:	Blood Sugar:
Temperature:	Oxygen Saturation:

DOCTOR VISITS

Test Ordered	Test Results

Prescription(s), Vitamins & Supplements

Name	Dosage	Duration

Notes:

DOCTOR VISITS

44

Doctor's Name	
Doctor's Office	
Telephone	
Date	Time
Reason for Visit	
Question(s) to Ask	
Doctor's Diagnose/ Feedback	
Prescribed Treatment	

Weight:	Blood Pressure:
Heart Rate:	Blood Sugar:
Temperature:	Oxygen Saturation:

DOCTOR VISITS

Test Ordered	Test Results

Prescription(s), Vitamins & Supplements

Name	Dosage	Duration

Notes:

DOCTOR VISITS

Doctor's Name	
Doctor's Office	
Telephone	
Date	Time
Reason for Visit	
Question(s) to Ask	
Doctor's Diagnose/ Feedback	
Prescribed Treatment	

Weight:	Blood Pressure:
Heart Rate:	Blood Sugar:
Temperature:	Oxygen Saturation:

DOCTOR VISITS

Test Ordered	Test Results

Prescription(s), Vitamins & Supplements

Name	Dosage	Duration

Notes:

DOCTOR VISITS

Doctor's Name	
Doctor's Office	
Telephone	

Date		Time	

Reason for Visit	
Question(s) to Ask	
Doctor's Diagnose/ Feedback	
Prescribed Treatment	

Weight:		Blood Pressure:	
Heart Rate:		Blood Sugar:	
Temperature:		Oxygen Saturation:	

DOCTOR VISITS

Test Ordered	Test Results

Prescription(s), Vitamins & Supplements

Name	Dosage	Duration

Notes:

DOCTOR VISITS

Doctor's Name	
Doctor's Office	
Telephone	
Date	Time
Reason for Visit	
Question(s) to Ask	
Doctor's Diagnose/ Feedback	
Prescribed Treatment	

Weight:	Blood Pressure:
Heart Rate:	Blood Sugar:
Temperature:	Oxygen Saturation:

DOCTOR VISITS

Test Ordered	Test Results

Prescription(s), Vitamins & Supplements

Name	Dosage	Duration

Notes:

DOCTOR VISITS

Doctor's Name	
Doctor's Office	
Telephone	
Date	Time
Reason for Visit	
Question(s) to Ask	
Doctor's Diagnose/ Feedback	
Prescribed Treatment	

Weight:	Blood Pressure:
Heart Rate:	Blood Sugar:
Temperature:	Oxygen Saturation:

DOCTOR VISITS

Test Ordered	Test Results

Prescription(s), Vitamins & Supplements

Name	Dosage	Duration

Notes:

DOCTOR VISITS

Doctor's Name	
Doctor's Office	
Telephone	
Date	Time
Reason for Visit	
Question(s) to Ask	
Doctor's Diagnose/ Feedback	
Prescribed Treatment	

Weight:	Blood Pressure:
Heart Rate:	Blood Sugar:
Temperature:	Oxygen Saturation:

DOCTOR VISITS

Test Ordered	Test Results

Prescription(s), Vitamins & Supplements

Name	Dosage	Duration

Notes:

DOCTOR VISITS

Doctor's Name	
Doctor's Office	
Telephone	
Date	Time
Reason for Visit	
Question(s) to Ask	
Doctor's Diagnose/ Feedback	
Prescribed Treatment	

Weight:	Blood Pressure:
Heart Rate:	Blood Sugar:
Temperature:	Oxygen Saturation:

DOCTOR VISITS

Test Ordered	Test Results

Prescription(s), Vitamins & Supplements

Name	Dosage	Duration

Notes:

DOCTOR VISITS

Doctor's Name	
Doctor's Office	
Telephone	
Date	Time
Reason for Visit	
Question(s) to Ask	
Doctor's Diagnose/ Feedback	
Prescribed Treatment	

Weight:	Blood Pressure:
Heart Rate:	Blood Sugar:
Temperature:	Oxygen Saturation:

DOCTOR VISITS

Test Ordered	Test Results

Prescription(s), Vitamins & Supplements

Name	Dosage	Duration

Notes:

DOCTOR VISITS

Doctor's Name	
Doctor's Office	
Telephone	
Date	Time
Reason for Visit	
Question(s) to Ask	
Doctor's Diagnose/ Feedback	
Prescribed Treatment	
Weight:	Blood Pressure:
Heart Rate:	Blood Sugar:
Temperature:	Oxygen Saturation:

DOCTOR VISITS

Test Ordered	Test Results

Prescription(s), Vitamins & Supplements

Name	Dosage	Duration

Notes:

DOCTOR VISITS

Doctor's Name	
Doctor's Office	
Telephone	
Date	Time
Reason for Visit	
Question(s) to Ask	
Doctor's Diagnose/ Feedback	
Prescribed Treatment	

Weight:	Blood Pressure:
Heart Rate:	Blood Sugar:
Temperature:	Oxygen Saturation:

DOCTOR VISITS

Test Ordered	Test Results

Prescription(s), Vitamins & Supplements

Name	Dosage	Duration

Notes:

DOCTOR VISITS

Doctor's Name	
Doctor's Office	
Telephone	
Date	Time
Reason for Visit	
Question(s) to Ask	
Doctor's Diagnose/ Feedback	
Prescribed Treatment	

Weight:	Blood Pressure:
Heart Rate:	Blood Sugar:
Temperature:	Oxygen Saturation:

DOCTOR VISITS

Test Ordered	Test Results

Prescription(s), Vitamins & Supplements

Name	Dosage	Duration

Notes:

DOCTOR VISITS

Doctor's Name	
Doctor's Office	
Telephone	
Date	Time
Reason for Visit	
Question(s) to Ask	
Doctor's Diagnose/ Feedback	
Prescribed Treatment	

Weight:	Blood Pressure:
Heart Rate:	Blood Sugar:
Temperature:	Oxygen Saturation:

DOCTOR VISITS

Test Ordered	Test Results

Prescription(s), Vitamins & Supplements

Name	Dosage	Duration

Notes:

DOCTOR VISITS

Doctor's Name	
Doctor's Office	
Telephone	
Date	Time
Reason for Visit	
Question(s) to Ask	
Doctor's Diagnose/ Feedback	
Prescribed Treatment	

Weight:	Blood Pressure:
Heart Rate:	Blood Sugar:
Temperature:	Oxygen Saturation:

DOCTOR VISITS

Test Ordered	Test Results

Prescription(s), Vitamins & Supplements

Name	Dosage	Duration

Notes:

DOCTOR VISITS

Doctor's Name	
Doctor's Office	
Telephone	

Date		Time	

Reason for Visit	
Question(s) to Ask	
Doctor's Diagnose/ Feedback	
Prescribed Treatment	

Weight:		Blood Pressure:	
Heart Rate:		Blood Sugar:	
Temperature:		Oxygen Saturation:	

DOCTOR VISITS

Test Ordered	Test Results

Prescription(s), Vitamins & Supplements

Name	Dosage	Duration

Notes:

DOCTOR VISITS

Doctor's Name	
Doctor's Office	
Telephone	
Date	Time
Reason for Visit	
Question(s) to Ask	
Doctor's Diagnose/ Feedback	
Prescribed Treatment	

Weight:	Blood Pressure:
Heart Rate:	Blood Sugar:
Temperature:	Oxygen Saturation:

DOCTOR VISITS

Test Ordered	Test Results

Prescription(s), Vitamins & Supplements

Name	Dosage	Duration

Notes:

DOCTOR VISITS

Doctor's Name	
Doctor's Office	
Telephone	
Date	Time
Reason for Visit	
Question(s) to Ask	
Doctor's Diagnose/ Feedback	
Prescribed Treatment	

Weight:	Blood Pressure:
Heart Rate:	Blood Sugar:
Temperature:	Oxygen Saturation:

DOCTOR VISITS

Test Ordered	Test Results

Prescription(s), Vitamins & Supplements

Name	Dosage	Duration

Notes:

DOCTOR VISITS

Doctor's Name	
Doctor's Office	
Telephone	
Date	Time
Reason for Visit	
Question(s) to Ask	
Doctor's Diagnose/ Feedback	
Prescribed Treatment	

Weight:	Blood Pressure:
Heart Rate:	Blood Sugar:
Temperature:	Oxygen Saturation:

DOCTOR VISITS

Test Ordered	Test Results

Prescription(s), Vitamins & Supplements

Name	Dosage	Duration

Notes:

DOCTOR VISITS

Doctor's Name	
Doctor's Office	
Telephone	

Date		Time	

Reason for Visit	
Question(s) to Ask	
Doctor's Diagnose/ Feedback	
Prescribed Treatment	

Weight:		Blood Pressure:
Heart Rate:		Blood Sugar:
Temperature:		Oxygen Saturation:

DOCTOR VISITS

Test Ordered	Test Results

Prescription(s), Vitamins & Supplements

Name	Dosage	Duration

Notes:

DOCTOR VISITS

Doctor's Name	
Doctor's Office	
Telephone	
Date	Time
Reason for Visit	
Question(s) to Ask	
Doctor's Diagnose/ Feedback	
Prescribed Treatment	

Weight:	Blood Pressure:
Heart Rate:	Blood Sugar:
Temperature:	Oxygen Saturation:

DOCTOR VISITS

Test Ordered	Test Results

Prescription(s), Vitamins & Supplements

Name	Dosage	Duration

Notes:

DOCTOR VISITS

Doctor's Name	
Doctor's Office	
Telephone	
Date	Time
Reason for Visit	
Question(s) to Ask	
Doctor's Diagnose/ Feedback	
Prescribed Treatment	

Weight:	Blood Pressure:
Heart Rate:	Blood Sugar:
Temperature:	Oxygen Saturation:

DOCTOR VISITS

Test Ordered	Test Results

Prescription(s), Vitamins & Supplements

Name	Dosage	Duration

Notes:

DOCTOR VISITS

Doctor's Name	
Doctor's Office	
Telephone	
Date	Time
Reason for Visit	
Question(s) to Ask	
Doctor's Diagnose/ Feedback	
Prescribed Treatment	

Weight:	Blood Pressure:
Heart Rate:	Blood Sugar:
Temperature:	Oxygen Saturation:

DOCTOR VISITS

Test Ordered	Test Results

Prescription(s), Vitamins & Supplements

Name	Dosage	Duration

Notes:

DOCTOR VISITS

Doctor's Name	
Doctor's Office	
Telephone	
Date	Time
Reason for Visit	
Question(s) to Ask	
Doctor's Diagnose/ Feedback	
Prescribed Treatment	

Weight:	Blood Pressure:
Heart Rate:	Blood Sugar:
Temperature:	Oxygen Saturation:

DOCTOR VISITS

Test Ordered	Test Results

Prescription(s), Vitamins & Supplements

Name	Dosage	Duration

Notes:

DOCTOR VISITS

Doctor's Name	
Doctor's Office	
Telephone	
Date	Time
Reason for Visit	
Question(s) to Ask	
Doctor's Diagnose/ Feedback	
Prescribed Treatment	

Weight:	Blood Pressure:
Heart Rate:	Blood Sugar:
Temperature:	Oxygen Saturation:

DOCTOR VISITS

Test Ordered	Test Results

Prescription(s), Vitamins & Supplements

Name	Dosage	Duration

Notes:

DOCTOR VISITS

Doctor's Name	
Doctor's Office	
Telephone	
Date	Time
Reason for Visit	
Question(s) to Ask	
Doctor's Diagnose/ Feedback	
Prescribed Treatment	

Weight:	Blood Pressure:
Heart Rate:	Blood Sugar:
Temperature:	Oxygen Saturation:

DOCTOR VISITS

Test Ordered	Test Results

Prescription(s), Vitamins & Supplements

Name	Dosage	Duration

Notes:

DOCTOR VISITS

Doctor's Name	
Doctor's Office	
Telephone	
Date	Time
Reason for Visit	
Question(s) to Ask	
Doctor's Diagnose/ Feedback	
Prescribed Treatment	

Weight:	Blood Pressure:
Heart Rate:	Blood Sugar:
Temperature:	Oxygen Saturation:

DOCTOR VISITS

Test Ordered	Test Results

Prescription(s), Vitamins & Supplements

Name	Dosage	Duration

Notes:

DOCTOR VISITS

Doctor's Name	
Doctor's Office	
Telephone	
Date	Time
Reason for Visit	
Question(s) to Ask	
Doctor's Diagnose/ Feedback	
Prescribed Treatment	

Weight:	Blood Pressure:
Heart Rate:	Blood Sugar:
Temperature:	Oxygen Saturation:

DOCTOR VISITS

Test Ordered	Test Results

Prescription(s), Vitamins & Supplements

Name	Dosage	Duration

Notes:

DOCTOR VISITS

Doctor's Name	
Doctor's Office	
Telephone	
Date	Time
Reason for Visit	
Question(s) to Ask	
Doctor's Diagnose/ Feedback	
Prescribed Treatment	

Weight:	Blood Pressure:
Heart Rate:	Blood Sugar:
Temperature:	Oxygen Saturation:

DOCTOR VISITS

Test Ordered	Test Results

Prescription(s), Vitamins & Supplements

Name	Dosage	Duration

Notes:

DOCTOR VISITS

Doctor's Name	
Doctor's Office	
Telephone	
Date	Time
Reason for Visit	
Question(s) to Ask	
Doctor's Diagnose/ Feedback	
Prescribed Treatment	

Weight:	Blood Pressure:
Heart Rate:	Blood Sugar:
Temperature:	Oxygen Saturation:

DOCTOR VISITS

Test Ordered	Test Results

Prescription(s), Vitamins & Supplements

Name	Dosage	Duration

Notes:

DOCTOR VISITS

Doctor's Name	
Doctor's Office	
Telephone	
Date	Time
Reason for Visit	
Question(s) to Ask	
Doctor's Diagnose/ Feedback	
Prescribed Treatment	

Weight:	Blood Pressure:
Heart Rate:	Blood Sugar:
Temperature:	Oxygen Saturation:

DOCTOR VISITS

Test Ordered	Test Results

Prescription(s), Vitamins & Supplements

Name	Dosage	Duration

Notes:

DOCTOR VISITS

Doctor's Name	
Doctor's Office	
Telephone	
Date	Time
Reason for Visit	
Question(s) to Ask	
Doctor's Diagnose/ Feedback	
Prescribed Treatment	

Weight:	Blood Pressure:
Heart Rate:	Blood Sugar:
Temperature:	Oxygen Saturation:

DOCTOR VISITS

Test Ordered	Test Results

Prescription(s), Vitamins & Supplements

Name	Dosage	Duration

Notes:

DOCTOR VISITS

Doctor's Name	
Doctor's Office	
Telephone	
Date	Time
Reason for Visit	
Question(s) to Ask	
Doctor's Diagnose/ Feedback	
Prescribed Treatment	

Weight:	Blood Pressure:
Heart Rate:	Blood Sugar:
Temperature:	Oxygen Saturation:

DOCTOR VISITS

Test Ordered	Test Results

Prescription(s), Vitamins & Supplements

Name	Dosage	Duration

Notes:

DOCTOR VISITS

Doctor's Name	
Doctor's Office	
Telephone	
Date	Time
Reason for Visit	
Question(s) to Ask	
Doctor's Diagnose/ Feedback	
Prescribed Treatment	

Weight:	Blood Pressure:
Heart Rate:	Blood Sugar:
Temperature:	Oxygen Saturation:

DOCTOR VISITS

Test Ordered	Test Results

Prescription(s), Vitamins & Supplements

Name	Dosage	Duration

Notes:

NOTES:

NOTES:

NOTES:

NOTES:

ADDRESS BOOK

PRIMARY CARE PHYSICIAN

Name

Telephone

Address

DENTIST

Name

Telephone

Address

OB-GYN

Name

Telephone

Address

EYE DOCTOR

Name

Telephone

Address

SPECIALIST ....

Name

Telephone

Address

SPECIALIST ....

Name

Telephone

Address

SPECIALIST ....

Name

Telephone

Address

SPECIALIST ....

Name

Telephone

Address

Printed in Great Britain
by Amazon